UNVEILING THE POWER

OF

MORINGA LEAVES

Unlocking Natures Green Secret A Journey to Revitalise Your Health and Energy

Charles Shakespeare

Table of Content

Introduction

The remarkable nutritional content and many uses of moringa leaves, sometimes known as "drumstick leaves" or "miracle leaves," have garnered much attention in recent times. The attention on moringa leaves is well-deserved in this age of growing health awareness and sustainable living, as it opens up a world of lucrative potential in a variety of businesses.

Supercharged Nutrition: Moringa's extraordinary nutritional profile is the main factor that draws people to it. Moringa leaves are an incredible source of vital nutrients since they are loaded with vitamins, minerals, and antioxidants. A single serving has a good quantity of calcium, potassium, iron, vitamin C, and vitamin A. Moringa's high nutrient content makes it an excellent complement to diets across the globe, helping to treat widespread nutritional deficits.

Business Cultivation: The cultivation of moringa is among its most profitable uses. Moringa trees are a lucrative and sustainable crop since they grow quickly, can withstand a variety of climates, and need little water. Farmers and entrepreneurs alike are investigating the financial possibilities of growing moringa for a range of uses, from domestic use to export.

Wellness and Health Advantages: The market for goods containing moringa is being driven by the health advantages of moringa leaves. Because of the leaves' anti-inflammatory, antibacterial, and antiviral qualities, they have been utilised for centuries. The health and wellness sector has seen a rise in moringa supplements, teas, and powders as contemporary research supports these claims, resulting in the creation of a lucrative market niche.

Delicious Foods: Moringa leaves are a culinary treat as well as a nutritious treasure. These leaves provide flavour and nourishment to a variety of meals with their mild, earthy taste. Chefs and food aficionados are using moringa leaves in their creations, which is expanding options in the culinary world, from salads to soups and smoothies.

Outside the Consumption: Moringa is used for purposes outside of the kitchen. The process of extracting the medicinal properties of moringa has resulted in the creation of oils, supplements, and cosmetics products. Because of its moisturising and anti-aging qualities, moringa oil—which is derived from the seeds—is becoming more and more well-liked, opening up a sizable market for the skincare and cosmetics sectors.

Sustainable Farming: Because of its adaptability to a variety of climates and capacity to increase soil fertility, moringa is an important component of sustainable agriculture. Its profitability is further increased by the leaves' use as a natural fertiliser and cattle feed, which draws in ecologically conscientious farmers and enterprises.

Strategies for Marketing: A thorough strategy is needed to sell moringa products in an effective manner. Effective marketing tactics entail informing customers about the whole benefits of integrating moringa into their life, from stressing its nutritional advantages to showcasing its adaptability in a range of sectors. Campaigns on social media, partnerships with health influencers, and presenting success stories are all important components of a strong marketing strategy.

Compliance with Regulations: It's important to navigate regulatory systems, just as in any new sector. Building confidence with stakeholders and customers requires adhering to strict rules regarding agriculture, food safety, and quality assurance. To build a strong basis for their businesses, entrepreneurs in the moringa industry must make an investment in comprehending and abiding by these rules.

Difficulties and Their Remedies: Despite the enormous potential for profit in the moringa sector, there are obstacles to overcome. These might include problems finding high-quality seeds, keeping up regular growing techniques, or surviving market rivalry. Proactive measures, on the other hand, may assist in overcoming these obstacles. Some of these include forming alliances with dependable suppliers, putting sustainable agricultural techniques into place, and encouraging innovation.

Result: The discovery of the nutritional value of moringa leaves also represents a doorway to lucrative business endeavours in other industries. Entrepreneurs, farmers, and health enthusiasts are realising moringa's many uses, turning it from a traditional cure to a worldwide sensation. A symbol of both economic possibility and nutritional richness, moringa is becoming more and more associated with sustainable living and holistic well-being.

Chapter 1:

Uncovering Nature's Nutritious Wonder

When it comes to superfoods, moringa leaves are a veritable nutritional wonder. The Moringa tree, which is native to regions of Africa, Asia, and Latin America, has long been valued for its abundance of nutrients and therapeutic qualities. It is clear that moringa leaves have the power to completely transform our understanding of health and wellbeing as we set out to investigate their nutritional benefits.

The Nutrient-Rich Profile of Moringa: An Extensive Analysis

The remarkable nutritional profile of moringa, which makes it a powerhouse of vital vitamins and minerals, is the main reason for its popularity. Vitamin A from moringa leaves is abundant and significantly improves immune system and eye health. They also include vitamin C, which is well-known for its antioxidant qualities that help the body fight free radicals. Vitamin E is another component that supports healthy skin and general wellbeing.

In moringa leaves, minerals including calcium, potassium, and iron are plentiful. Iron is essential for avoiding anaemia, potassium helps heart health by controlling blood pressure, and calcium is necessary for keeping healthy bones and teeth. This thorough analysis demonstrates why moringa is often referred to as a "multivitamin in a leaf."

Using Moringa to Meet Dietary Requirements for Protein

Moringa leaves are a useful option for those on plant-based diets or looking for other sources of protein. Surprisingly, moringa is a complete protein, which means that it has every important amino acid required for the body to operate properly. Because of this, moringa is a great option for vegans, vegetarians, and anybody trying to increase the variety of proteins in their diet.

In addition to helping with muscle growth, moringa's high protein concentration helps with weight control by encouraging a sensation of fullness. Moringa is a nutrient-dense, sustainable protein source that is becoming more and more popular as plant-based protein demands grow.

Supercharged with Antioxidants: Fighting Oxidative Stress

A common antecedent to many chronic illnesses is oxidative stress, which is caused by an imbalance in the body's levels of antioxidants and free radicals. Because of their strong antioxidant qualities, moringa leaves are essential for scavenging free radicals and reducing oxidative damage.

Quercetin, chlorogenic acid, and beta-carotene are among the antioxidants included in moringa that help to reduce inflammation and cell damage. Frequent moringa intake may be seen as a preventative step to strengthen the body's defences against oxidative stress, which will promote long-term health and lower the risk of age-related illnesses.

Moringa and Immune Support: Using Nature to Boost Wellness

Moringa leaves are a natural ally in the quest for strong immune health. Moringa's vitamin, mineral, and antioxidant combinations work together to fortify the immune system. Specifically, vitamin C promotes the development of white blood cells, which are vital for warding off infections and diseases. More than just vitamins, moringa boosts immunity because it has substances like beta-glucans that activate immunological responses. Adding moringa leaves to meals is becoming a proactive, all-encompassing strategy for general well being as people look for natural methods to strengthen their immune systems.

Regulation of Blood Sugar: The Effect of Moringa on the Management of Diabetes

A potential natural method of controlling blood sugar levels is provided by moringa leaves, which address the worldwide health challenge of the incidence of diabetes. According to studies, chemicals found in moringa may help reduce blood sugar by improving insulin sensitivity and delaying the body's absorption of sugar.

Incorporating moringa leaves into one's diet may help those with diabetes or those at risk maintain stable blood sugar levels. This potential not only takes care of a serious health concern, but it also establishes moringa as a significant dietary ingredient in the expanding functional food sector.

Heart Health: The Beneficial Effects of Moringa on the Heart

Since cardiovascular illnesses continue to be the world's leading cause of death, many people's top priority is maintaining good heart health. Moringa leaves have a number of beneficial effects on cardiovascular health. The potassium concentration lowers the risk of hypertension and related cardiovascular problems by assisting in blood pressure regulation.

Moringa's remarkable capacity to reduce cholesterol levels is another benefit. A healthy cholesterol level may be maintained by including moringa leaves in the diet, since high cholesterol is a major risk factor for heart disease. The incorporation of moringa becomes more pertinent as knowledge about heart health prevention strategies increases.

Moringa: A Calcium-Rich Remedy for Bone Health

Keeping bones strong and healthy is crucial for general health, particularly as people age. Because of their high calcium content, moringa leaves are essential for maintaining bone health. Consuming enough calcium is essential to preventing fractures and diseases like osteoporosis.

When dairy intake is restricted, moringa becomes a great plant-based calcium supply. This feature presents moringa as a sustainable and all-inclusive answer to a range of nutritional demands in addition to filling a dietary gap.

Intestinal Health: The Beneficial Effects of Fibre from Moringa

The high fibre content of moringa leaves contributes to its digestive effects. In order to keep the digestive tract functioning normally, encourage frequent bowel movements, and avoid constipation, dietary fibre is crucial. Because moringa leaves are an innate supply of soluble and insoluble fibre, they support digestive health in general.

While insoluble fibre gives stool more volume and facilitates its easy transit through the digestive system, soluble fibre found in moringa helps control cholesterol and blood sugar levels. Moringa's high fibre content makes it a useful meal for gut health, particularly as digestive health continues to get attention in the wellness community.

Moringa: An Added Nutrient for Lactation and Pregnancy

A well-rounded, nutrient-dense diet is essential during pregnancy and breastfeeding because of the increased nutritional needs of these times. With so many vitamins and minerals, moringa leaves provide a natural boost to address these higher nutritional needs.

Packed with iron, calcium, and vitamin A, moringa promotes the growth of the pregnancy and keeps the mother and baby healthy throughout nursing. Moringa is being recognized as a beneficial dietary supplement for pregnant moms and those going through the postpartum phase as understanding of the significance of maternal nutrition rises.

Recovery and Athletic Performance: Moringa as a Natural Supplement

In the realm of fitness and sports, maximising performance and accelerating recuperation are critical. Because of its high nutritional content and adaptogenic qualities, moringa leaves are a great natural supplement for athletes looking to get an advantage over their training schedules.

Moringa's protein content aids in the growth and repair of muscles, while its antioxidants help to lower oxidative stress and inflammation brought on by strenuous exercise. Moringa may be added to smoothies before a workout or to meals afterward, making it a useful addition to any athlete's or fitness enthusiast's diet.

Nourishing the Brain with Moringa for Cognitive Health

With increasingly busy lives, cognitive health is becoming a significant issue. Moringa leaves provide a natural way to fuel the brain. Packed with neuroprotective and antioxidant properties, moringa may improve cognitive function and lower the incidence of neurodegenerative illnesses.

Moringa contains compounds with antioxidant and anti-inflammatory properties, such as quercetin and chlorogenic acid

Chapter 2:

Revealing the Profit Potential of Moringa Plantation

Growing moringa is more than simply a farming endeavour—it's a successful enterprise that integrates business savvy, sustainability, and nutrition. The moringa plant becomes an advantageous crop for both farmers and business owners as the need for organic, nutrient-dense foods grows. In this investigation, we examine the factors—such as its adaptability, low resource needs, and wide range of market prospects—that have contributed to the success and sustainability of moringa cultivation.

Adaptability of Moringa: Succeeding in Various Settings

Moringa's extraordinary flexibility is one of the main characteristics that make it profitable to cultivate. Because moringa can grow in a variety of conditions, including tropical and desert ones, it is a practical plant to cultivate all over the world. This flexibility reduces the dangers brought on by erratic weather patterns and enables farmers in different areas to benefit economically from the production of moringa.

Furthermore, the cultivation potential of moringa is further enhanced by its capacity to thrive in unfavourable soil conditions. Moringa is hardy enough to thrive in regions where other crops fail, giving farmers a chance to make use of otherwise unused land.

High Yield and Quick Growth: A Formula for Success in Agriculture

Because moringa grows so quickly and produces so much, cultivating it is a worthwhile undertaking. Moringa trees may mature quickly; in fact, they typically do so in the first year after planting. With many harvests possible in a single year due to this rapid growth cycle, the possibility for money creation is greatly increased.

The economic worth of moringa is enhanced by its large output of leaves, pods, and seeds. Moringa is a profitable crop that may be grown on a small or large scale due to the number of raw materials it produces, which can be used to make value-added products or picked for fresh consumption.

Minimum Resources Needed: Optimising Profit Margins

The minimal resource needs of moringa cultivation make it an economical and productive agricultural paradigm. Because moringa trees can survive with little water, they are a good choice for areas where water is scarce. Because of its innate water efficiency, farmers may maximise their profit margins by minimising production expenses and lessening their negative environmental effects.

Additionally, the resilience of moringa to diseases and pests reduces the need for heavy pesticide usage, making agriculture more economical and sustainable. Growing in popularity among environmentally concerned customers and companies, moringa stands out as a crop that adheres to sustainable and eco-friendly agriculture techniques, as the globe moves toward these practices.

Varieties of Market Prospects: Not Just Fresh Produce

Growing moringa is profitable even outside of the conventional fresh product market. Moringa leaves, pods, and seeds are versatile and provide a variety of commercial prospects. Moringa has several uses, ranging from goods for health and wellness to the food and beverage sector.

The increasing demand in the health and wellness industry for supplements, teas, and powders based on moringa presents an opportunity for entrepreneurs. Because of their abundant nutrient profile, leaves are a popular choice for customers looking for natural, plant-based substitutes in nutritional supplements.

The culinary community also loves moringa for its distinct taste and health advantages. A niche market for culinary goods infused with moringa is emerging as a result of chefs and food aficionados using the leaves of the plant in a range of recipes. By allowing cultivators to investigate several income sources, this diversity of market options lessens their reliance on a particular market niche.

Moringa Oil: Getting Into the Profitable Skincare and Beauty Sector

The priceless moringa oil, a major component in the profitable skincare and cosmetics sector, is derived from the seeds of the moringa tree. Because of its anti-inflammatory, anti-aging, and moisturising qualities, moringa oil is highly sought-after as a component in cosmetic formulas.

Farmers may generate extra revenue by growing moringa for oil extraction, as consumers are becoming more interested in eco-friendly and natural healthcare products. The growing inclination of the cosmetic business towards plant-based products presents moringa oil as a lucrative commodity, hence fostering a positive correlation between agriculture and beauty.

Using Moringa for Sustainable Agriculture: An Eco-Friendly and Profitable Method

Moringa's profitability is further increased by its use in sustainable agriculture. The natural fertiliser that the moringa tree's leaves provide the earth with vital minerals. Moringa is a cover crop that improves the general health of agricultural ecosystems by reducing soil erosion and inhibiting the development of weeds. Increased crop yields in following plantings, less dependence on synthetic fertilisers, and greater soil fertility are all benefits seen by farmers including moringa into their crop rotation plans. This environmentally friendly strategy not only helps the environment but also presents moringa growers as guardians of environmentally friendly agriculture, attracting environmentally concerned customers and improving financial performance.

Marketing Techniques for Moringa Products: Narrating the Sustainability and Health Story

More than emphasising the nutritional advantages of moringa products are needed for effective marketing; a captivating narrative about health and sustainability is also necessary. Customers who are looking for wholesome goods that also happen to be ecologically conscientious will find a narrative that is created when they are informed about the process from agriculture to consumption.

Establishing a robust brand presence for moringa products may be achieved via strategic partnerships with health and wellness influencers, social media campaigns, and packaging that tells a narrative. Stressing the ethical and sustainable components of moringa production enhances brand value and draws in a rising customer base that places a high value on environmental responsibility, ethical sourcing, and wellness.

Successful Moringa Businesses: Case Studies

Analysing case studies of successful moringa enterprises offers insightful information about the tactics and procedures that support their development. Examining these success stories, whether they are small-scale farms that have successfully entered the local market or bigger businesses with a worldwide presence, enables prospective growers and entrepreneurs to get insight into the critical elements that contribute to the profitability of the moringa sector.

Case studies highlight the many strategies that might result in success in the moringa industry, from creative product creation to efficient supply chain management. Newcomers to the sector may make well-informed judgments and strategically position their initiatives for development and sustainability by learning from the experiences of others.

Future Developments and Innovations in the Moringa Sector: Leading the Way

Maintaining profitability requires keeping up with emerging trends and advances, just as in any dynamic sector. The destiny of the moringa industry is always being shaped by continuing research and technical breakthroughs. By examining the possible effects of new developments, including creative product formulations, improved farming techniques, or technology innovations, growers and business owners may establish themselves as industry leaders.

Staying ahead of the curve guarantees that firms can adjust to changing customer expectations and industry norms, whether it's implementing sustainable packaging solutions, adopting precision agricultural methods, or investigating new products based on moringa. In a competitive and evolving business, moringa ventures is positioned as leaders thanks to proactive engagement with emerging trends.

Quality Control and Regulatory Compliance: Creating Market Trust

A vital component of guaranteeing the moringa industry's long-term prosperity is navigating the regulatory environment. Building confidence with stakeholders and customers requires strict adherence to agricultural laws, food safety standards, and quality assurance procedures. Comprehending and adhering to these guidelines not only protects the status of moringa enterprises but also guarantees the security and

Chapter 3:

Moringa's Health and Wellness Advantages

With everyone seeking the best possible health, moringa has gained attention as the "miracle tree." Moringa is a plant with a wide range of nutritional and therapeutic uses that go far beyond just its vivid green leaves. In this investigation, we break down the mysteries of moringa's ascent to prominence as a formidable superfood and examine its revolutionary effects on overall health, ranging from boosting immunity to reducing inflammation.

Energy-Dense Essence: Moringa as a Whole Food Supplement

The unmatched nutritional richness of moringa is the foundation of its health benefits. The leaves of the moringa plant are a powerful source of vitamins, minerals, and antioxidants. Significant concentrations of vitamin A, vitamin C, calcium, potassium, and iron are present in this botanical treasure trove, which provides a complete dietary supplement that meets a range of nutritional demands.

Moringa's rich vitamin content supports a healthy immune system, eyesight, and skin renewal. In the meanwhile, the vital minerals are crucial for heart health, blood oxygen delivery, and bone health. Moringa appears as a practical and organic means of supplying a range of nutrients necessary for general health and well-being to the diet.

Energy-Dense Essence: Moringa as a Whole Food Supplement

Because of its exceptional antioxidant capacity, moringa is a valuable tool in the fight against ageing and illness. Many antioxidants found in moringa tree leaves, such as beta-carotene, chlorogenic acid, and quercetin, actively fight free radicals in the body.

As a result of regular body functions and outside stimuli, free radicals may harm cells and accelerate the ageing process as well as a number of illnesses. These free radicals are neutralised by the antioxidants in moringa, extending life and avoiding cellular harm. Frequent moringa ingestion turns into a proactive strategy for bolstering the body's resistance to oxidative stress.

Destroyer of Inflammation: The Anti-Inflammatory Properties of Moringa

Many contemporary illnesses, including autoimmune disorders and cardiovascular problems, are caused by chronic inflammation. Because of its strong anti-inflammatory qualities, moringa is becoming more and more popular as a natural way to reduce inflammation and improve general health.

Studies have shown that compounds like the isothiocyanates present in moringa have anti-inflammatory properties. Including moringa in the diet might help lower inflammation and hence relieve some of the symptoms related to inflammatory diseases. Because of its anti-inflammatory properties, moringa may be a useful part of a comprehensive strategy for controlling long-term health problems.

Immune Support: The Function of Moringa in Boosting the Body's Defences

The body's first line of defence against infections and illnesses is a strong immune system. Rich in nutrients that strengthen the immune system, moringa leaves are essential for bolstering the body's defences. Specifically, vitamin C is necessary for the development and operation of white blood cells, which are the main actors in the immune response.

Frequent moringa ingestion strengthens the immune system and may lessen the severity and frequency of illnesses. With more people placing a higher priority on preventative healthcare, moringa becomes a convenient and natural way to boost immunological resilience.

Regulation of Blood Sugar: The Effect of Moringa on the Management of Diabetes

Interest in natural methods of controlling blood sugar levels has increased due to the rise of diabetes, and moringa has shown to be a potential ally in this field. Studies indicate that blood sugar regulation may be aided by the bioactive components found in moringa, such as chlorogenic acid.

By including moringa in their diet, those with diabetes or those at risk may help to keep their blood sugar levels steady. This possibility not only takes care of a serious health concern, but it also fits in with the increasing demand from consumers for functional meals that improve overall health.

Enhanced Cardiovascular Health: Beneficial Impacts of Moringa on Heart Function

Heart health is critical, especially considering the increased prevalence of cardiovascular illnesses. Moringa leaves have a number of beneficial effects on cardiovascular health. Because moringa contains potassium, it lowers the risk of hypertension and related cardiovascular problems by regulating blood pressure.

Furthermore, moringa offers an additional degree of cardiovascular protection by lowering cholesterol. The use of moringa in the diet may help to maintain healthy cholesterol levels, since high cholesterol is a major risk factor for heart disease. Moringa is a natural and nutritious supplement to a heart-healthy lifestyle, especially as people become more conscious of their heart health.

Bone Health Booster: The Benefits of Moringa for Strong Bones

Keeping bones strong and healthy is essential for general health, particularly as people age. Because of their remarkable calcium concentration, moringa leaves are a useful ally in the promotion of bone health. Consuming enough calcium is essential to preventing fractures and diseases like osteoporosis.

Moringa offers a plant-based substitute for dairy in areas where dairy use is restricted to increase calcium intake. This feature presents moringa as a sustainable and all-inclusive answer to a range of nutritional demands in addition to filling a dietary gap.

Healthy Digestive System: The Fiber-Rich Support of Moringa for Gut Health

The high fibre content of moringa leaves aids in digestion and provides a natural, plant-based remedy for preserving intestinal health. Dietary fibre is essential for maintaining a healthy digestive tract, encouraging regular bowel movements, and avoiding constipation.

Soluble and insoluble fibre found in moringa leaves support healthy digestion. While insoluble fibre gives faeces more volume and facilitates its easy transit through the digestive system, soluble fibre helps control cholesterol and blood sugar levels. Moringa's fibre-rich composition puts it as a functional meal for gut health as digestive health gets attention in the wellness community.

Moringa during Lactation and Pregnancy: Nourishing Mother and Child

Mothers have increased nutritional needs throughout pregnancy and nursing, therefore what they eat is important for the mother's health as well as the health of the growing child. With so many vitamins and minerals, moringa leaves provide a natural boost to address these higher nutritional needs.

Packed with iron, calcium, and vitamin A, moringa promotes the growth of the pregnancy and keeps the mother and baby healthy throughout nursing. Moringa is being recognized as a beneficial dietary supplement for pregnant moms and those going through the postpartum phase as understanding of the significance of maternal nutrition rises.

Recovery and Athletic Performance: Moringa as Nature's Exercise Supplement

In sports and fitness, it's critical to maximise performance and minimise recuperation time. Because of its high nutritional content and adaptogenic qualities, moringa leaves are a great natural supplement for athletes looking to get an advantage over their training schedules.

Moringa's protein content aids in the growth and repair of muscles, while its antioxidants help to lower oxidative stress and inflammation brought on by strenuous exercise. Moringa becomes a useful addition to athletes' and fitness fanatics' diet regimens when added to smoothies made before workouts or meals eaten afterward. It increases endurance and speeds up recovery.

Moringa for Mental Well-Being: Fueling the Brain for Extended Life

With increasingly busy lives, cognitive health is becoming a significant issue. Moringa leaves provide a natural way to fuel the brain. Packed with neuroprotective and antioxidant properties, moringa may improve cognitive function and lower the incidence of neurodegenerative illnesses.

Substances such as qu

Chapter 4:

Moringa in Culinary Delights Enhancing Recipes and Culinary Uses

Not only is moringa found in teas and capsules, but it is also well praised for its outstanding nutritional profile. Its adaptability also reaches into the kitchen, where its vivid green leaves and pods offer a fascinating touch to a wide range of recipes. We delve into the culinary joys of moringa in this investigation, revealing inventive culinary uses and inventive dishes that increase taste while also using the remarkable nutritional advantages of this plant.

Moringa Leaves: A Culinary Gem Packed with Nutrients

Prior to digging into particular recipes, it's important to acknowledge the main attraction: moringa leaves. These vitamin, mineral, and antioxidant-rich leaves give food a subtle earthy taste while also packing a nutritious punch. Because of their adaptability, moringa leaves may be used in a wide range of food preparations, including soups and salads.

Pasta Moringa Pesto: A Combination of Tastes and Nutrients

Making a bright green moringa pesto is one creative approach to add moringa to food treats. To make a nutrient-rich pesto sauce, blend fresh moringa leaves with garlic, basil, pine nuts, Parmesan cheese, and olive oil. Combine it with whole-grain pasta to create a filling and tasty dish that combines traditional and healthful elements.

With its vibrant green colours, this moringa pesto pasta not only brightens up the eating experience but also gives a traditional meal a new dimension of flavour and nutrition. Moringa boosts the vitamin and mineral richness of the meal, transforming it from a basic pasta recipe into a gastronomic celebration of well-being.

Smoothies with Moringa Infusions: A Refreshing Nutrient Boost

Smoothies are a delicious way for those who want to include moringa in their morning or snack routine. Mix moringa leaves into a delicious, nutrient-rich smoothie by blending them with fruits like bananas, berries, and a little coconut water.

This smoothie, which has been infused with moringa, is a handy way to get the nutritional advantages of moringa without sacrificing taste. Smoothies' adaptability enables people to try out various fruit combinations, customising the recipe to suit individual tastes and taking advantage of the moringa's abundant nutritional content.

Quinoa Salad with Moringa Spices: A Wholesome Powerhouse

Salads become a blank canvas for creative cooking, and adding moringa to a basic salad transforms it into a nutritious powerhouse. Mix cooked quinoa with a variety of fresh veggies, bell peppers, cucumbers, and cherry tomatoes. Add some moringa leaves for a nutritious and colourful pop.

The tastes are enhanced without overwhelming the inherent health of moringa, thanks to a simple dressing made with olive oil, lemon juice, and a little amount of salt. This quinoa salad with moringa spices is a visual treat that also demonstrates how versatile moringa is when it comes to improving the nutritional value of commonplace foods.

Moringa-infused Soups: Comforting Bowls Packed with Nutrients

Soups are a cosy go-to dinner when the weather cools. Moringa adds taste and nutrients to soups in a way that blends in effortlessly. Whether included into a traditional vegetable soup or a filling lentil stew, moringa leaves enrich the liquid with an abundance of vitamins and minerals.

Soups with moringa extract are quite versatile. There are many variations, from creamy moringa spinach soup to spicy moringa lentil soup. With the healthful benefits of moringa, these soups feed the body as well as the spirit.

Guacamole with Moringa Infusion: A Modern Take on a Classic Dip

The addition of moringa makes guacamole—known for its creamy avocado base—even more alluring. For a distinct and nutrient-rich guacamole, mash ripe avocados and combine them with chopped tomatoes, onions, cilantro, lime juice, and a dash of moringa powder.

This guacamole with a hint of moringa adds a nutritional boost in addition to a vivid green colour that enhances the flavour. Avocados provide beneficial lipids, while moringa adds a range of vitamins and antioxidants. A traditional dip is elevated to a gastronomic experience that pleases the palate and the health-conscious mind thanks to a combination of flavours.

Hummus with Moringa Infusion: A Complete Dip with a Unique Taste

Addition of moringa boosts the nutritional value of hummus, a common dish in many homes. Mix together chickpeas, tahini, garlic, lemon juice, and a good pinch of moringa powder to make a hummus that is enriched with moringa powder and packed full of nutrients.

This moringa hummus turns into a multipurpose spread that goes well with fresh veggies, whole-grain crackers, and sandwiches. The nuttiness of the chickpeas and the earthy tones of the moringa combine to create a harmonic combination that improves the nutritional profile of this popular dip.

Healthy Twist on Sweet Indulgences: Desserts Infused with Moringa

Who said desserts had to be delicious and healthful? Rich in minerals and with a gentle green colour, moringa is a wonderful addition to sweet delights. Add moringa powder to smoothie bowls, energy bites, and even muffins and pancakes for dessert.

Because of its subtle taste, moringa may be used in a variety of dessert dishes without taking over from the sweetness. These desserts—banana bread with moringa infusion or moringa bliss balls—become guilt-free treats that provide a delicious way to saute sweet cravings and take advantage of moringa's health advantages.

Elixirs rich in nutrients: Drinking Beverages laced with Moringa

Drinks provide yet another way to include moringa into delicious dishes. For instance, the earthy undertones of moringa leaves combined with hot water make a calming and nourishing beverage known as moringa tea. Squeezing in a little honey or lemon improves the taste profile without compromising the nutritious value.

Additionally, moringa may be used in cold drinks like green smoothies or iced tea with moringa extract. These reviving mixtures support the rising trend towards healthy drink alternatives by providing a hydrated and nutrient-rich substitute for sugary drinks.

Result: Moringa Brings Nutritional Excellence and Culinary Creativity Together

In summary, the culinary benefits of moringa go much beyond the conventional limits of superfood usage. Moringa leaves, pods, and powder are versatile enough to be used in a wide range of inventive culinary applications, from savoury recipes to sweet treats and everything in between. A culinary jewel, moringa turns common meals into nutrient-rich works of art as foodies and health-conscious customers enjoy the marriage of taste and nutrition. Eaten in a robust soup, a colourful salad, or as a dessert, moringa encourages people to experience the flavour of health and wellness one delicious meal at a time.

Chapter 5:

Extracting Moringa's Healing Potential Supplements and Extracts

The plant known technically as Moringa , or moringa, has drawn a lot of interest due to its extraordinary therapeutic qualities. For decades, traditional medicine has used moringa, a plant rich in vitamins, minerals, and amino acids, to treat many ailments. Its wide range of bioactive ingredients, which include beta-carotene, chlorogenic acid, and quercetin, may help it recover.

Studies have shown that moringa has antibacterial, antioxidant, and anti-inflammatory properties, which validate its traditional usage. Its anti-inflammatory qualities aid with ailments like arthritis, and its antioxidant content lowers the chance of developing chronic illnesses by battling oxidative stress. Moringa is a useful tool in natural medicine as its antibacterial qualities also aid in its capacity to combat illnesses.

Types of Moringa Extracts: A key factor in maximising the therapeutic benefits of moringa is the extraction procedure. The concentrations of bioactive chemicals produced by various extraction techniques differ. The conventional approach of extracting water is economical, but it may not remove all useful substances. A wide range of bioactive compounds are known to be preserved using the more advanced and effective method of ethanol extraction. Although it guarantees excellent purity, supercritical CO_2 extraction is a sophisticated process with greater operating expenses.

It is essential for individuals wishing to join the moringa supplement sector to comprehend these extraction techniques. Every strategy has benefits and drawbacks that affect the finished product's quality and standing in the market.

Well-liked Supplements for Moringa: As more people look for natural and holistic health remedies, the demand for supplements containing moringa has increased. Popular forms that satisfy various tastes include oils, powders, and capsules. Convenience and accurate dosage are two features that draw in health-conscious customers to moringa capsules. For those who want flexibility, moringa powder can simply be used in a variety of dishes. Because of its high antioxidant content, moringa oil is used in skincare and haircare products.

Investigating these supplement kinds gives business owners a better understanding of client preferences and enables them to customise their product offerings to satisfy a range of market needs.

Starting a Successful Business: A calculated strategy is needed to break into the moringa supplement industry. It's critical to comprehend the current trends in the herbal supplement business. Moringa has a lot of promise because of the trend toward natural and plant-based medicines worldwide. But it's important to navigate the regulatory environment. Getting the required certifications guarantees that the product meets health requirements and is of high quality.

Finding premium sources for Moringa leaves is essential to starting a successful company. Developing a rapport with dependable suppliers and making sure that sustainable practices are followed are important factors in the venture's overall success. In order to ensure that their Moringa extracts are effective, entrepreneurs need to also take into account aspects like growth techniques, harvesting procedures, and post-harvest treatment.

Marketing Strategies: In order to effectively sell Moringa supplements, awareness must be raised and a strong brand image must be developed. Education is essential; people must be aware of the advantages of moringa and the reasons it stands out from the competition in the supplement industry. Reaching a larger audience is facilitated by using influencers, social media, and online platforms.

Partnerships with shops and associations with health and wellness professionals may increase exposure. In a visually competitive industry, packaging design that highlights the natural and premium attributes of Moringa products helps draw customers.

Case Studies: Analysing successful companies in the morning sector offers prospective company owners insightful information. Businesses that have overcome obstacles, put successful marketing plans into place, and maintained product quality may teach us about long-term, steady development. Case studies highlight how crucial it is to be flexible, creative, and aware of what customers want in a market that is always changing.

Examining the paths taken by well-established companies that sell moringa supplements may provide insight into best practices, possible hazards, and long-term success in this booming sector. These examples might serve as a source of inspiration for entrepreneurs looking to improve their company strategy and increase the likelihood that they will have a positive market effect.

Chapter 6:

Moringa in Cosmetics and Skincare Revealing the Lucrative Prospects

The cosmetics and skincare sector has seen a paradigm change in favour of sustainable and natural products in recent years. With its wide range of bioactive chemicals and nutrient-rich profile, moringa has become a prominent player in this field. Investigating the use of moringa into skincare and cosmetics reveals a plethora of lucrative prospects.

- **The Powerhouse of Nutrients:**

Boasting critical minerals, vitamins A, C, and E, and amino acids, moringa is a nutritional powerhouse. These components nourish the skin and provide a natural way to encourage a glowing, healthy complexion. Making use of moringa's natural nutritional advantages gives beauty products a distinctive marketing point.

- **Youthful Skin with Antioxidant Elixir:**

Because of its high antioxidant content, moringa is an effective defence against oxidative stress, which is a major cause of early ageing. By battling free radicals, moringa is added to skincare formulas to help minimise the look of wrinkles and fine lines. Moringa-infused beauty products are becoming a popular option for those looking for anti-aging treatments that work.

- **Marvel's Anti-Inflammatory:**

Because of its anti-inflammatory qualities, moringa is a great choice for treating eczema and acne as well as calming inflamed skin. Beauty products that use the anti-inflammatory properties of moringa provide a mild but effective skincare solution. Customers who value goods that support skin health without harsh chemicals are drawn to this.

- **Natural Hydration:**

The oil derived from the seeds of the moringa plant is well known for its ability to moisturise. It works well as an ingredient in moisturisers, creams, and serums because of its non-greasy, lightweight texture. Deep hydration is provided by beauty products containing moringa, leaving the skin smooth and refreshed. This hydration feature meets consumer demand for skincare products that put moisture retention and skin health first.

- **The Trend of Sustainable Beauty:**

Sustainable and environmentally friendly beauty options are attracting more and more customers. Moringa's quick growth, low water needs, and adaptability to a variety of climes make it a perfect fit for this trend. Beauty companies that use moringa may benefit from the eco-aware customer base that is looking for goods that have a beneficial environmental effect.

- **Brand Story and Market Differentiation:**

Brands trying to stand out in a crowded industry might find a differentiator by including moringa into their cosmetic products. A captivating narrative is created by telling the tale of moringa's natural origin, traditional use, and advantages supported by research. In addition to adding value to the brand, this narrative strategy appeals to customers who desire authenticity in their skincare selections.

- **Versatility and Global Appeal:**

Moringa is popular around the world since it is used in many traditional and cultural medical practices. By creating solutions that address a variety of skin types and issues, beauty firms may reach a large spectrum of consumers. Because of its adaptability, moringa may be used to create skincare products for a variety of skin types, including acne-prone and anti-aging.

- **Transparency and Consumer Education:**

Encouraging customers to learn about the skincare advantages of moringa promotes brand loyalty and trust. Credibility is increased by open communication on the source of ingredients, extraction techniques, and the research behind moringa's therapeutic benefits. Companies that engage in consumer education cultivate an informed clientele that recognizes the benefits of beauty products containing moringa.

Chapter 7:

Moringa Oil: Seizing a Profitable Chance

In the cosmetic and wellness sector, businesses are considering moringa oil as a profitable opportunity as the demand for natural and sustainable beauty products continues to increase. This oil, which is made from the seeds of the Moringa tree, is becoming more and more well-known for its many uses and advantages for the skin and hair. Examining the potential of moringa oil reveals a multitude of chances for those looking to make a successful business in the expanding natural beauty solutions sector.

Moringa Oil's Beauty: The abundance of vitamins A, C, and E, as well as important fatty acids and antioxidants, found in moringa oil are among its many health benefits. Because of its ability to provide moisture, anti-aging benefits, and defence against free radicals, it is a very potent component for skincare products. These innate traits may be used by entrepreneurs venturing into the moringa oil sector to produce high-end cosmetic products.

Skin Care Supplement: Moringa oil is a lightweight, readily absorbable moisturiser that works wonders for a variety of skin types. Entrepreneurs may meet the increasing demand from consumers for natural substitutes for traditional moisturisers by creating skincare products including face oils, serums, and creams. Moringa oil's commercial appeal is increased by presenting it as a nourishing elixir for attractive skin.

Organic Anti-Aging Remedies: Moringa oil is a very effective anti-aging remedy because of its antioxidant-rich content. Fine lines, wrinkles, and other indications of ageing may be targeted by beauty products containing moringa oil. By creating serums, eye creams, and anti-wrinkle treatments that capitalise on the restorative properties of moringa oil, business owners may capitalise on the anti-aging industry.

Revolution in Hair Care: The health benefits of moringa oil for hair have been shown; they go beyond skincare benefits. It strengthens and nourishes hair strands as a deep conditioner, encouraging a glossy and healthy mane. To capitalise on the need for natural hair care solutions, entrepreneurs should investigate producing hair care products like conditioners, masks, and oils.

Appeal to the Environment: Because of its quick growth and capacity to adapt to many conditions, moringa trees are considered to be an ecologically benign resource. Businesses that use moringa oil in their cosmetics might draw in customers who care about the environment by highlighting the plant's eco-friendliness. This is in line with the expanding movement for ethical and sustainable cosmetic options.

Worldwide Market Coverage: Because of its widespread popularity, moringa oil gives business owners access to a variety of international marketplaces. Creating products that target certain issues with the skin and hair guarantees a large customer base. Because moringa is used in traditional medicine throughout cultures, beauty firms may develop products that appeal to customers across the world who are looking for natural, culturally relevant solutions.

Marketing Strategies for Education: In order to join the Moringa oil industry successfully, one must use marketing methods that are focused on education. Entrepreneurs may emphasise the advantages of moringa oil supported by research, outlining its ingredients and how it takes care of different beauty issues. Consumer education establishes the company as an expert on natural beauty solutions and fosters consumer trust.

Transparency and Quality Assurance: Transparency and quality control are essential for enterprises to flourish in the cutthroat cosmetics sector. Credibility is established by making the source, extraction process, and purity of Moringa oil in beauty products evident. Brand loyalty is fostered by visible labelling and certifications, which boost customer trust.

Chapter 8:

Harnessing Moringa for Sustainable Agriculture

With its many advantages that go far beyond its customary usage as a medical plant, moringa emerges as a potent ally in the field of sustainable agriculture. Farmers and entrepreneurs alike are realising that moringa has the potential to revolutionise farming methods, advance environmental sustainability, and provide financial rewards. This article explores how using moringa for sustainable agriculture may lead to a green revolution that benefits the environment and the economy.

Marvel of Agroforestry: Moringa, often called the "miracle tree" or "drumstick tree," grows well in agroforestry systems. Because of its quick growth, especially in dry environments, it's a great choice for forestry projects. By growing high-value Moringa products, integrating Moringa into agroforestry not only helps to conserve soil but also creates a second source of revenue.

Erosion control and soil enrichment: The capacity of moringa to increase soil fertility is one of its amazing qualities. Because of its deep taproot system, the plant increases water absorption and decreases erosion by breaking up compacted soil. When mulched or mixed with the soil, moringa leaves serve as a natural fertiliser, adding vital nutrients to the soil. Because of its ability to both improve soil quality and reduce erosion, moringa is an invaluable tool for sustainable agricultural methods.

Livestock Feed Rich in Nutrients: In addition to being healthy for people, moringa leaves provide cattle with nutrient-rich feed. Planters of Moringa may be established by business people interested in sustainable agriculture as a dependable and wholesome feed for animals. This enhances the health of the cattle and helps create an agricultural ecology that is more self-sufficient and sustainable.

Biodiesel Potential: Oil from moringa seeds may be extracted and used to make biodiesel. This creates opportunities for the generation of bioenergy, providing a sustainable substitute for traditional fossil fuels. To help renewable energy projects and lessen reliance on non-renewable resources, sustainable agricultural entrepreneurs should investigate producing biodiesel from Moringa oil.

Crops That Use Less Water: Compared to many other crops, moringa is renowned for its remarkable water efficiency and requires very little irrigation. This is especially important in areas where water is scarce. Farmers may maximise water use and contribute to resilient water management and climate change adaptation by using moringa into their agricultural methods.

Farmers' Income Diversification: Moringa cultivation offers farmers a variety of revenue streams. The leaves, seeds, and pods of the Moringa plant may be used to make a variety of goods, including oils, cosmetics, and nutritional supplements. Businesses that work with nearby farmers to include moringa into their farming methods improve communities' economic standing and promote sustainable agriculture.

Champion of Carbon Sequestration: Through its ability to absorb carbon dioxide during photosynthesis, moringa contributes to carbon sequestration. Initiatives for sustainable agriculture help to mitigate climate change by encouraging the development of moringa. This environmental advantage supports a more sustainable and greener future and is in line with international initiatives to cut greenhouse gas emissions.

Education for Community Empowerment: For moringa to be successfully included into sustainable agriculture, community engagement and education are necessary. In order to educate farmers about the benefits of growing Moringa, sustainable farming methods, and other financial prospects, entrepreneurs may play a critical role. Providing communities with information guarantees the sustainability and long-term viability of agricultural projects based on moringa.

Chapter 9:

Promoting Moringa Products Fostering Success in a Developing Market

Entrepreneurs hoping to profit from this growing sector must adopt successful marketing techniques as moringa's health advantages and many uses become more well-known. Here's a comprehensive look into lucrative marketing strategies made just for Moringa goods, ranging from supplements to cosmetics and beyond.

1.Instructional Materials as a Foundation: Promote moringa products as educational resources rather than merely commodities. Provide educational materials that inform readers on the history, nutritional value, and science behind the health advantages of moringa. Educative movies, infographics, and blog entries increase credibility and engage readers while also gaining their confidence.

2. Showcasing Eco-Friendly and Sustainable Practices: Emphasise Moringa's eco-friendly properties. Highlight how Moringa supports ethical and sustainable consumer decisions, from its adaptability to many climates to its low water needs. Customers are looking for items that have less of an influence on the environment, and moringa's sustainable characteristics fit well with this idea.

3. Using Branding to Tell Stories: Craft an engaging brand story about Moringa. Tell the tale of its historical applications, cultural relevance, and farm-to-product transformation. Authentic tales captivate consumers, and incorporating the historical significance of moringa into your branding creates an emotional connection that extends beyond the purchase.

4. Certifications and Quality Control: Reassure customers on the quality of your morning offerings. Acquire the necessary certifications for fair trade, organic, or non-GMO operations. To reassure consumers about the product's legitimacy and compliance with industry standards, be sure to prominently display these certificates on packaging and promotional materials.

5. Collaborations with Influencers: To increase your reach, work with wellness and health influencers. Collaborate with influencers that connect with Moringa's natural and holistic approach. Influencers have the ability to provide real content, tell their stories about using Moringa products, and recommend your company to their interested audience.

6. Diverse Product Lines for a Range of Customers:
Acknowledge moringa's adaptability and expand your
offerings. Adapt to varying customer demands and
tastes with a range of goods, including skincare,
haircare, and culinary items. By doing this, you broaden
your consumer base and establish your company as the
go-to source for everything related to moringa.

7. Participate on Social Media Sites: Create a lively
online presence on various social media sites. Share
visually engaging articles, client testimonials, and
updates regarding Moringa's advantages. Promote
user-generated content by putting up challenges or
competitions. In order to create a feeling of community
around your business, interact with your audience via
direct messages and comments.

**8. Working Together with Wellness and Health
Professionals:** Form alliances with experts in nutrition,
health, and wellbeing, or even with chefs who can attest
to the advantages of moringa. Their knowledge gives
your company legitimacy, and their endorsements may
sway a larger audience looking for reliable industry
voices.

9. Testimonials and Reviews from Customers:
Put client endorsements and reviews front and centre in
your marketing collateral. Positive comments increase
confidence and act as social confirmation of the benefits
of moringa. Urge contented clients to provide their

experiences in the form of written evaluations, images, or videos.

10. Offline and Online Distribution Strategy:
Make the most out of your traditional and online distribution platforms. To increase your market reach, collaborate with wellness centres, health food shops, and e-commerce platforms. Enticing packaging and well-positioned physical displays help to increase the exposure of your Moringa goods overall.

A comprehensive strategy including education, sustainability, genuineness, and strategic alliances is necessary for the effective marketing of moringa products. By putting these tactics into practice, business owners can successfully negotiate the competitive environment and position their Moringa products for long-term development and financial success in a market that is ravenous for healthy, natural solutions.

Chapter 10:

Case Studies: Revealing the Triumphs of Robust Moringa Enterprises

Entrepreneurship focused on this adaptable plant has blossomed, and moringa has emerged as a star player in the health and wellness space. Analysing these Moringa companies' success stories offers insightful information about successful tactics, obstacles surmounted, and room for expansion in this rapidly growing sector.

1. Kuli Kuli: Bringing Moringa to the Level of Superfood: Kuli Kuli, which Lisa Curtis founded in 2011, has pioneered new developments in the moringa sector. The company's main goal is to produce food items made from moringa, especially powders and bars for energy. Moringa was cleverly positioned by Kuli Kuli as a superfood, with a focus on sustainability and nutritional richness. In addition to guaranteeing a steady supply of premium Moringa, the firm promoted community development by forming alliances with smallholder farmers across the world. The secret of Kuli Kuli's success is its dedication to quality, moral sourcing, and creative product creation.

2. Moringa Well-Being: Linking Conventional Knowledge with Contemporary Health: Moringa Wellness, a firm formed by Dr. Howard W. Fisher, has carved a niche by blending ancient knowledge with contemporary health solutions. Motivated by a love of traditional medicine, Moringa Wellness provides a selection of supplements made from moringa. The company's success stems from its thorough research, which makes sure that its products follow the traditional applications of moringa while also complying with scientific standards. By emphasising instruction, Moringa Wellness has effectively conveyed the health advantages of the plant and developed a devoted following of clients who appreciate the incorporation of age-old knowledge into modern wellness regimens.

3. Veritable Moringa: From Farm to Glamor:
Kwami Williams and Emily Cunningham co-founded True Moringa, which is notable for its dedication to ethical and environmental operations. The firm has expanded into the beauty sector by introducing skincare items in addition to producing supplements based on moringa. The secret to True Moringa's success is their vertically integrated supply chain, which gives them complete control over the whole manufacturing process—from farming to processing. The brand capitalised on the natural beauty trend by introducing

Moringa oil into skincare products, which appealed to customers looking for cruelty-free and environmentally friendly options.

4. Empowering Local Farmers with Majestic Moringa: The company Majestic Moringa, which was founded in a rural area, is a prime example of the transformational potential of moringa farming. Majestic Moringa was established by a group of regional farmers working with agricultural specialists, with an emphasis on organic Moringa growing and the manufacturing of a range of Moringa products. Majestic Moringa was able to reduce poverty and foster community development in addition to making a substantial profit by providing the local population with information and sustainable farming methods.

5. MoringaConnect: Leveraging Innovation to Increase Impact: Kwami Williams and Emily Cunningham's startup, MoringaConnect, is a prime example of using innovation to advance social good. The firm created a novel processing method to generate Moringa oil in addition to producing items based on the moringa plant. MoringaConnect promotes economic emancipation and guarantees a stable supply chain by creating a network of smallholder growers in Ghana. The key factors contributing to MoringaConnect's success are its inventiveness, community involvement, and resolve to bring about constructive social and economic change.

Key Learnings and Conclusions:

- **Diversification is Essential**:
Profitable moringa companies often expand the range of products they provide by partnering with companies in the food, supplement, cosmetic, and other sectors.

- **Sustainability Promise:**
The incorporation of ethical and sustainable methods, such as fair trade alliances and environmentally friendly projects, enhances the prosperity and favourable reputation of moringa enterprises.

- **Community Engagement and Empowerment:**
Companies that actively support and empower farmers and other local groups not only guarantee a steady supply chain but also advance social progress.

- **Innovation Drives Growth**:
Businesses that embrace innovation, whether it is in product creation, processing methods, or supply chain management, set themselves up for long-term success in the cutthroat moringa market.

Ultimately, these case studies provide light on the many avenues for success within the Moringa industry. Entrepreneurs may learn a great deal from these successful businesses and use creative approaches to overcome obstacles, take advantage of market trends, and support the industry's continuous expansion.

Chapter 11:

Innovations and Future Trends in the Moringa Sector: Crossing the Green Frontier

Future developments and breakthroughs that will reshape the landscape are expected to be exciting as the moringa sector continues to flourish due to its widely acknowledged health advantages and diverse range of uses. With moringa taking centre stage in a number of industries, consumers, farmers, and entrepreneurs may look forward to a more sustainable and greener future. A sneak peek at the new developments and trends that will shape the morning industry's future is provided here.

1. Sophisticated Processing Methods for Improved Products: The development of sophisticated processing methods is about to transform the creation of new Moringa products. Technological advancements in extraction techniques, such microencapsulation and nanoencapsulation, will increase the bioavailability of the bioactive components in moringa. As a consequence, customers will be able to completely benefit from the health advantages of the plant and the supplements will be more effective and readily absorbed.

2. Foods with Functions and Fortified Goods: Expect to see a sharp increase in the use of moringa in functional meals and goods that have been fortified. Moringa will become a common element in goods that seek to provide consumers not just nourishment but also a natural boost of vital nutrients, such as energy bars, drinks, and snacks. This pattern is in line with consumers' increasing desire for nutrient-dense, functional foods.

3. Culinary Applications of Innovation: The culinary community is about to use moringa in novel ways. In a variety of cuisines, chefs and food aficionados will experiment with using moringa leaves, powder, and oil. The plant's distinct taste profile and nutritional richness will spur culinary innovation and contribute to a gastronomic revival in everything from gourmet meals to sauces infused with moringa.

4. Moringa Supplements and Tailored Nutrition: Personalised nutrition is the way of the future, and moringa supplements are no different. Anticipate customised Moringa products that address certain health requirements. This trend, which includes tailored dose forms and supplement mixes, shows how committed the business is to meeting the needs and tastes of individual consumers.

5. Blockchain Technology for Transparency in the Supply Chain: Transparency in the supply chain is becoming a top priority for customers. The use of blockchain technology will be essential to guaranteeing the validity and traceability of goods containing moringa. Customers will have access to comprehensive information on the path taken by Moringa products from farm to table, fostering trust in their quality and ethical source.

6. Solutions for Biodegradable Packaging: Customer preferences are influenced by sustainability. There will be a movement in the moringa sector toward environmentally friendly packaging options. Packaging that is compostable and biodegradable will become standard, signifying a dedication to lessening environmental effect and supporting the larger eco-conscious movement.

7. Informational Digital Platforms for Customers: The growth of the moringa industry will make digital platforms essential for instruction. Businesses will use technology to educate customers about the health advantages of moringa, share recipes, and provide customised health insights. This will include interactive websites and mobile applications. Digital channels will help create a Moringa community by bringing customers and brand ambassadors together.

8. Novelties in Genetics and Agronomy: Research on genetics and agronomy will advance to produce Moringa varieties that are tailored to certain uses and climates. This will improve overall agricultural sustainability, disease resistance, and crop output. More advancements in precision farming, such as intelligent irrigation and soil monitoring, will boost the productivity of moringa plantations.

9. Moringa in Personal Care and Cosmetics: The demand for goods infused with moringa will soar in the beauty and personal care sector. A crucial component of natural and sustainable beauty formulas is moringa oil, which is well-known for its advantages for skincare. Because of its moisturising and anti-aging qualities, moringa will become a highly sought-after ingredient in skincare and haircare products.

10. Untapped Bioactive Compound Research: Research will continue to reveal previously unknown bioactive chemicals in moringa, hence increasing the plant's potential uses. Investigating the less well-known components of moringa scientifically will result in the creation of new products with particular health-promoting qualities. Innovation, sustainability, and a holistic approach to health and wellbeing will define the moringa industry's future.

The green frontier of the moringa industry will be shaped in large part by entrepreneurs and stakeholders who adopt these new trends and developments, providing customers with a wide choice of goods that help create a more sustainable and healthy future.

Chapter 12:

Regulatory Compliance and Quality Assurance: Pillars of Product Integrity and Consumer Trust

In the dynamic landscape of industries, regulatory compliance and quality assurance stand as fundamental pillars ensuring the safety, efficacy, and integrity of products. From pharmaceuticals to food, cosmetics to technology, adherence to regulatory standards and robust quality assurance processes is paramount. This is particularly crucial in industries like health supplements, where consumer trust is closely tied to the safety and efficacy of products. Let's delve into the significance of regulatory compliance and quality assurance, their interplay, and the measures businesses take to meet these essential requirements.

1. Regulatory Compliance: Safeguarding Public Health and Market Integrity: Regulatory compliance refers to the adherence of businesses to laws, regulations, and standards set by government authorities or industry bodies. In the health supplement industry, regulatory compliance is overseen by agencies like the Food and Drug Administration (FDA) in the United States, the European Medicines Agency (EMA) in Europe, and various national health agencies worldwide. These regulatory frameworks ensure that products meet established safety, quality, and labelling standards, protecting public health and fostering fair competition in the market.

2. Quality Assurance: A Holistic Approach to Product Excellence:** Quality assurance is a comprehensive system of processes, checks, and measures designed to ensure that products meet predefined quality standards. In the health supplement industry, this involves rigorous testing of raw materials, manufacturing processes, and finished products to guarantee consistency, purity, and potency. Quality assurance is not only about meeting regulatory requirements but also about delivering products that meet or exceed customer expectations.

3. Interplay Between Regulatory Compliance and Quality Assurance: Regulatory compliance and quality assurance are interdependent facets of product development and distribution. While regulatory compliance sets the legal framework and minimum requirements, quality assurance goes beyond these standards to achieve excellence in product quality. Businesses that excel in quality assurance not only meet regulatory requirements but also establish a reputation for delivering high-quality, reliable products.

4. Ensuring Product Safety: One of the primary goals of both regulatory compliance and quality assurance is to ensure the safety of products. Rigorous testing for contaminants, proper handling of raw materials, adherence to Good Manufacturing Practices (GMP), and accurate labelling all contribute to minimising risks associated with health supplements. Meeting safety standards not only protects consumers but also shields businesses from legal liabilities.

5. Building Consumer Trust: Consumer trust is a precious commodity in any industry, and it is particularly vital in sectors that involve health and well-being. Demonstrating regulatory compliance and robust quality assurance practices builds trust by assuring consumers that products are safe, reliable, and meet or exceed established standards. This trust becomes a significant competitive advantage and fosters brand loyalty.

6. Navigating International Markets: For businesses operating in the global marketplace, understanding and complying with diverse regulatory frameworks is a complex but essential task. International markets may have different standards and requirements, necessitating a nuanced approach to regulatory compliance and quality assurance. Adapting products to meet these diverse standards opens up opportunities for businesses to expand their reach.

7. Investment in Research and Development: A commitment to quality assurance often involves a substantial investment in research and development. By staying ahead of scientific advancements and industry trends, businesses can proactively adapt their products to meet evolving regulatory standards and consumer expectations. This investment not only ensures compliance but also positions businesses at the forefront of innovation

8. Documentation and Record-Keeping: Robust documentation and record-keeping are integral to both regulatory compliance and quality assurance. Maintaining detailed records of manufacturing processes, testing results, and any deviations from standard procedures is essential for demonstrating due diligence. In the event of audits or inquiries, thorough documentation serves as evidence of a company's commitment to quality and compliance.

9. Continuous Improvement: Regulatory standards and consumer expectations evolve over time. Successful businesses view regulatory compliance and quality assurance as ongoing processes that require continuous improvement. Regular audits, feedback loops, and staying abreast of industry updates enable businesses to adapt and enhance their practices in response to changing conditions.

10. The Role of Technology: Technology plays a pivotal role in streamlining regulatory compliance and quality assurance processes. From advanced testing equipment to sophisticated data management systems, technology empowers businesses to conduct more accurate and efficient assessments. Automation of certain processes also reduces the likelihood of human error, enhancing the reliability of quality assurance measures.

In the intricate tapestry of industries, regulatory compliance and quality assurance emerge as essential threads that weave together the fabric of product integrity, consumer safety, and market trust. Successful businesses recognize the symbiotic relationship between these two pillars, viewing compliance not merely as a legal obligation but as an opportunity to showcase their commitment to excellence. By investing in quality assurance, businesses not only meet regulatory standards but also exceed them, paving the way for sustained success and enduring consumer confidence. As industries continue to evolve, the collaboration between regulatory bodies, businesses, and consumers will remain vital in shaping a landscape where products are not just compliant but consistently exceed expectations.

Chapter 13:

Overcoming Obstacles, Fostering Achievement: Remedies in Moringa Farming

Growing moringa, which is praised for its sustainabi ity and variety of uses, is not without its difficulties. Farmers who cultivate moringa have challenges that need for calculated solutions, ranging from insect control to climatic fluctuation. This essay examines the major obstacles that moringa farmers must overcome and offers creative ideas to open the door to successful and long-lasting production.

1. Adaptation to Change and Climate Sensitivity:
- **Difficulty:** Despite its reputation for flexibility, moringa can't grow to its full potential under harsh weather conditions like protracted droughts or severe rains.

- **Solution:** Farmers may lessen the effects of weather variations by putting climate-smart strategies into practice, including collecting rainwater, installing effective irrigation systems, and choosing Moringa types that are suited to the local area.

2. Management of Pests and Diseases:
- **Difficulty:** Aphids, caterpillars, and fungi are among the pests and diseases that may harm moringa plants and reduce crop productivity.

- **Remedy:** Reliance on chemical solutions is decreased by using integrated pest management (IPM) techniques such companion planting, natural predators, and biopesticides. Effective management of pests and diseases depends on early detection and routine monitoring.

3. Fertility and Soil Health:
- **Difficulty:** Strong Moringa growth depends on soil fertility, and ongoing cultivation may deplete soil nutrients.

- **Remedy:** Soil health is improved by using sustainable agricultural techniques including crop rotation, cover crops, and organic fertilising. Farmers may better customise fertiliser management to meet individual needs by regularly testing their soil.

4. Harvesting Procedures and Timing:
- **Difficulty:** For best quality and yield, choose the right time to harvest Moringa leaves, pods, or seeds.

- **Remedy:** Consistency in production is improved by using appropriate pruning methods and coordinating harvesting dates with the growth cycle of moringa. Farmworkers who participate in training programs are guaranteed to comprehend and adhere to proper methods for harvesting crops.

5. Seed Quality and Germination:

- **Difficulty:** Poor germination rates and inconsistent seed quality may make it difficult to successfully cultivate moringa.

- **Remedy:** Obtaining premium seeds from reliable vendors and carrying out germination assessments before sowing increase the probability of a successful establishment. Using seed priming methods improves the rate of germination.

6. Post-Harvest management and Storage:

- **Difficulty:** To maintain the nutritional value of moringa, careful post-harvest management is necessary due to its fragile leaves and pods.

- **Remedy:** Nutrient retention is ensured by using effective drying techniques, such as low-temperature drying or sun drying. Airtight containers and other suitable storage spaces protect Moringa products from moisture and deterioration.

7. Value Addition and Market Access:
- **Difficulty:** For small-scale farmers, it may be difficult to add value to their moringa products and get access to profitable markets.

- **Remedy:** Collective market access is made possible by establishing robust agricultural cooperatives or partnerships. Investigating value addition may improve a product's marketability and profitability. Examples of value addition include converting moringa into oils, powders, or cosmetics.

8. Education and Farmer Training:
- **Difficulty:** Farmers may not be well-versed in the best methods for growing moringa if they are not trained in them.

- **Remedy:** Putting money into farmer education initiatives, seminars, and extension services helps spread the word about sustainable agricultural methods, pest control, and ideal growing techniques. Farmers who are empowered make wise judgments and contribute to the sector's overall prosperity.

9. Sustainable Farming Certification:
- **Difficulty:** Maintaining certification requirements is necessary to meet the increasing demand for responsibly produced Moringa products.

- **Remedy:** Aiming for and receiving certifications such as Fair Trade or organic fits in with consumer preferences and builds trust. Using sustainable agricultural methods supports social responsibility and environmental preservation.

10. Policy Advocacy and Government Support:
- **Difficulty:** Farmers of moringa may face difficulties due to ambiguous agricultural regulations and a lack of government assistance.

- **Remedy:** Farmers and other industry participants may contact government officials to promote measures that will help the economy and environment by emphasising the advantages of growing moringa. Working together with agricultural extension services guarantees farmers have access to resources and current knowledge.

Even if growing moringa poses some difficulties, creative fixes and proactive approaches enable growers to get beyond roadblocks and foster success. Individual farm prosperity is bolstered by a resilient strategy that incorporates sustainable practices, ongoing learning, and industry partner engagement. This method also helps to the industry's overall development and sustainability in the moringa sector. Farmers of Moringa may successfully negotiate the difficulties of production, realise the enormous potential of the plant, and support a vibrant and successful agricultural industry by taking on these obstacles head-on.

Chapter 14:

Conclusion: Developing Self-Reliance with Moringa

Few crops have the same transformational potential in agriculture as moringa. Beneath its verdant foliage and densely packed seeds, there is a transformative agent inside it - a botanical energy that transcends farming and profoundly strengthens communities. As we approach to the end of our investigation into the significance of Moringa, it is clear that this extraordinary plant is more than simply a food source; it also serves as a catalyst for community empowerment and a signpost for a day when sustainability, health, and economic success will coexist.

1. Wellness and Health as Foundations: The unmatched nutritional profile of moringa is the foundation of its empowering properties. Moringa, being abundant in vitamins, minerals, and antioxidants, acts as a natural remedy for malnutrition and strengthens communities against health issues. Growing and eating moringa invigorates diets, providing nourishment to people and families as well as a preventative health strategy.

2. Moringa Enterprises Promote Economic Prosperity: Moringa provides the basis for sustainable lives, not just a crop. Communities may create economic possibilities by cultivating Moringa and producing value-added goods. Farmers who grow Moringa in a variety of climates and businesses who make health items and cosmetics are examples of how Moringa firms develop into economic engines that propel local wealth.

3. Sustainable Agriculture and Environmental Stewardship: The resilience and flexibility of moringa contribute to the sustainability of the ecosystem. Because of its soil-improving properties and capacity to flourish in a variety of climes, it is a champion of sustainable agriculture. Communities participate in ecologically aware agriculture by including Moringa into agricultural techniques, which promote biodiversity and soil health.

4. Knowledge Transfer and Educational Empowerment: With Moringa, the journey is about more than simply spreading seeds—it's about sowing knowledge. Transferring knowledge and education are essential to empowering communities. Farmers take on the role of stewards of their land with the help of cutting-edge methods and best practices. Workshops, courses, and cooperative projects provide a knowledge ecology in which the wisdom of growing Moringa is disseminated and preserved.

5. Enhancing Gender Equality and Empowering Women: The moringa plant is a symbol of female empowerment. In the processing and growing of moringa, women, who are often the backbone of agricultural communities, are essential. Gender equality advances as women discover chances for economic independence and communal leadership, from managing Moringa orchards to spearheading business projects.

6. Market Access and Worldwide Recognition:

Growing moringa provides doors to possibilities throughout the world and goes beyond local markets. Communities that use moringa have access to a global market of customers who are becoming more health-conscious. Communities are positioned to contribute to the greater story of sustainably and ethically derived goods as a result of the plant's widespread awareness.

7. Developing Resilience Despite Adversities:

Moringa empowers communities and makes them more resilient to adversity. Moringa becomes a resilient ally, providing answers to complex problems, whether it's solving nutritional inadequacies in disadvantaged communities or lessening the effects of climate change via its resilience.

8. History of Culture and Cuisine:

Moringa is more than simply a crop; it has a rich culinary and cultural history. Locals include moringa into customary dishes to retain cultural uniqueness and adopt contemporary health trends. As a link to sustainable practices and a source of pride in cultural history, the plant serves as a bridge between generations.

9. A Joint Approach to the Welfare of the Community: Using Moringa is a cooperative endeavor. Cooperation between farmers, business owners, researchers, and legislators is necessary to optimize the benefits of moringa for the welfare of local communities. Partnerships encourage creativity, information sharing, and the creation of long-term solutions that improve communities.

10. A Sustainable Heritage for Upcoming Generations: By embracing Moringa, communities plant the seeds for a sustainable future for coming generations. The long-lasting advantages of moringa are a legacy that is shared by families and communities, guaranteeing that the empowerment that this amazing plant started will endure and flourish.

Finally, moringa is shown as a plant that is not only amazing to look at but also a source of empowerment. It creates a fabric in which cultural diversity, economic success, environmental protection, and good health all come together. As communities all around the world embrace moringa, they set out on a path of empowerment, building a future in which this remarkable plant's leaves come to represent wealth, resilience, and well-being.

9 798875 834448